THE COMPLETE 2024 PRITIKIN DIET COOKBOOK FOR BEGINNERS

Delicious, Heart-Healthy Recipes for Weight Loss and Longevity with A Comprehensive Guide for Managing Diabetes

LUCKY WILSON

Table of Contents

WELCOME TO PRITIKIN DIET.........

INTRODUCTION

The Pritikin Diet is a low-fat, high-fiber diet that encourages the consumption of whole, natural foods. The diet was developed by Nathan Pritikin in the 1950s, and it has since become a popular dietary approach for weight loss and health improvement. The diet emphasizes the importance of consuming whole, natural foods, and discourages the consumption of processed and refined foods that are high in sugar, fat, and calories.

The History of the Pritikin Diet

The Pritikin Diet was developed by Nathan Pritikin, a businessman who was diagnosed with heart disease at a young age. Pritikin was determined to find a way to improve his health and, after conducting extensive research, he developed a low-fat, high-fiber diet that he believed could reverse heart disease. Pritikin adopted this diet himself and found that he was able to reduce the severity of his heart disease symptoms, and also lose weight. After seeing the benefits of his diet, Pritikin started sharing his knowledge with others, and the Pritikin Diet was born. The Pritikin Diet has become popular among people who want to improve their health and lose weight. The diet is based on the principle of consuming whole, natural foods that are low in fat and high in fiber. This means that the diet is rich in fruits, vegetables, whole grains, and lean proteins, which provide the body with the nutrients it needs to function properly.

Key Principles of the Pritikin Diet

The Pritikin Diet is based on several key principles, including:

• Eating whole, natural foods

• Consuming a variety of vegetables and fruits

• Getting enough fiber in your diet

• Reducing your intake of saturated fat and cholesterol

• Keeping your sodium intake low

Following these principles means that you will be consuming a lot of whole, natural foods, such as fruits, vegetables, whole grains, and lean meats. This means that you are getting the nutrients that your body needs, without consuming unnecessary calories, fat, or sugar. The Pritikin Diet also emphasizes the importance of exercise in maintaining good health. Regular exercise is an important part of the Pritikin Diet. Exercise helps to build muscle, burn fat, and improve cardiovascular health. The Pritikin Diet encourages people to engage in regular physical activity, such as walking, jogging, swimming, or cycling, for at least 30 minutes a day.

Foods to Eat and Avoid on the Pritikin Diet

On the Pritikin Diet, you should be eating a variety of foods that are good for your health. Some examples of foods that you should be eating include:

• Fruits, such as apples, bananas, berries, and oranges

• Vegetables, such as broccoli, spinach, carrots, and kale

• Whole grains, such as brown rice, quinoa, and whole wheat bread

• Lean proteins, such as chicken, turkey, and fish

• Low-fat dairy products, such as yogurt and milk

These foods are all low in fat and high in fiber, which makes them ideal for weight loss and good health. They are also rich in vitamins, minerals, and other nutrients that are essential for good health.

On the other hand, there are some foods that you should avoid when following the Pritikin Diet. These include:

• Foods that are high in saturated fat, such as butter, cream, and fatty cuts of meat

• Foods that are high in sugar, such as candy, cookies, and soda

• Foods that are high in sodium, such as processed foods, canned goods, and fast food

By avoiding these foods, you can improve your health and lose weight. The Pritikin Diet is a healthy and sustainable way to lose weight and improve your overall health. By following the principles of the diet, you can achieve your weight loss goals and improve your health and well-being.

Health Benefits of the Pritikin Diet

The Pritikin Diet has numerous health benefits. Some of the most significant benefits include:

1. Improved Heart Health: The Pritikin Diet is one of the best diets for heart health. It has been shown to lower cholesterol levels, reduce the risk of heart disease, and improve cardiovascular health. By following the Pritikin Diet, you can improve your heart health and reduce your risk of heart disease. One of the ways the Pritikin Diet improves heart health is by reducing the intake of saturated and trans fats. These types of fats can clog arteries and increase the risk of heart disease.

The Pritikin Diet encourages the consumption of healthy fats, such as those found in nuts, seeds, and fatty fish, which can help to reduce inflammation and improve heart health. In addition to improving heart health, the Pritikin Diet has also been shown to reduce inflammation throughout the body. Chronic inflammation is a major risk factor for heart disease, cancer, and other health complications. By reducing inflammation, the Pritikin Diet can help to improve overall health and reduce the risk of chronic diseases.

2. Weight Loss and Management: The Pritikin Diet is a great option for those who want to lose weight. It is low in calories, high in fiber, and promotes the consumption of whole, natural foods. This means that you can lose weight without feeling hungry or deprived.

Additionally, since the Pritikin Diet encourages the consumption of whole, natural foods, you are less likely to regain the weight once you have lost it. Research has shown that the Pritikin Diet can be more effective for weight loss than other popular diets, such as the Atkins Diet. This is likely due to the high fiber content of the Pritikin Diet, which helps to keep you feeling full and satisfied.

3. Enhanced Diabetes Control: The Pritikin Diet is particularly beneficial for those with diabetes. It has been shown to improve blood sugar control, reduce insulin resistance, and lower the risk of diabetes complications. By

following the Pritikin Diet, you can better manage your diabetes and reduce your risk of long-term health complications. The Pritikin Diet is low in simple carbohydrates and high in complex carbohydrates, which can help to regulate blood sugar levels. Additionally, the high fiber content of the diet can slow the absorption of glucose into the bloodstream, which can further help to regulate blood sugar levels.

4. Lowered Blood Pressure: High blood pressure is a major risk factor for heart disease. The Pritikin Diet has been shown to lower blood pressure, which reduces the risk of heart disease and other health complications. By following the Pritikin Diet, you can improve your blood pressure and overall health.

The Pritikin Diet is low in sodium and high in potassium, which can help to regulate blood pressure. Additionally, the diet encourages the consumption of whole, natural foods, which are generally lower in sodium than processed foods.

5. Reduced Cancer Risk: The Pritikin Diet has also been shown to reduce the risk of cancer. Since the diet encourages the consumption of whole, natural foods that

are rich in vitamins, minerals, and antioxidants, it helps to protect your body against the development of cancer cells. Research has shown that a diet high in fruits and vegetables can reduce the risk of several types of cancer, including lung, breast, and colon cancer. The Pritikin Diet is rich in fruits and vegetables, making it a great option for reducing cancer risk.

How the Pritikin Diet Promotes Weight Loss

The Pritikin Diet is effective for weight loss for several reasons.

1. Calorie Density and Portion Control: The Pritikin Diet is based on the principle of calorie density. This means that foods with a lower calorie density, such as fruits, vegetables, and whole grains, are more filling and can help you consume fewer calories overall. Additionally, the Pritikin Diet encourages portion control, which means that

you will be consuming smaller portions of food, but more frequently throughout the day.

2. High Fiber Intake: The Pritikin Diet is high in fiber, which can help you feel full and satisfied. Fiber also slows down the absorption of carbohydrates, which means that you will be less likely to experience spikes in blood sugar and insulin levels. By consuming more fiber, you can reduce your overall calorie intake and promote weight loss.

3. Low Fat Consumption: The Pritikin Diet is low in fat, which means that you will be consuming fewer calories overall. Additionally, since fat is more calorie-dense than other macronutrients, consuming less fat can help you lose weight more effectively. The Pritikin Diet encourages the consumption of healthy fats, such as those found in nuts, seeds, and fatty fish.

4. Regular Exercise and Physical Activity: The Pritikin Diet also encourages regular exercise and physical activity. Exercise can help you burn calories and promote weight loss. Additionally, exercise is important for overall health and can help you maintain your weight loss over time.

The Pritikin Food Pyramid

The Pritikin Food Pyramid emphasizes a diet rich in whole, unprocessed foods to promote health and longevity. At the base of the pyramid are vegetables, fruits, whole grains, and legumes, which should form the bulk of daily intake.

These foods are nutrient-dense, high in fiber, and low in calories, aiding in weight management and disease prevention. The next tier includes lean proteins such as fish, poultry, and plant-based proteins like tofu and beans, which support muscle maintenance and overall bodily functions. Dairy products are limited to low-fat options, focusing on moderation. Healthy fats, sourced from nuts, seeds, and avocados, are used sparingly to support cardiovascular health.

The top of the pyramid consists of foods to be consumed minimally, including refined grains, sweets, and high-fat, high-sodium processed foods. The Pritikin Food Pyramid encourages balanced nutrition and mindful eating to foster a healthy lifestyle.

Key Nutrients of Pritikin Diet and Their Roles

The Pritikin Diet emphasizes several key nutrients, each playing a vital role in promoting health and well-being:

1. Fiber: Found abundantly in vegetables, fruits, whole grains, and legumes, fiber aids in digestion, helps maintain healthy blood sugar levels, and supports weight management by promoting satiety.

2. Vitamins and Minerals: The diet is rich in vitamins A, C, E, and various B vitamins, as well as minerals like potassium, magnesium, and calcium. These nutrients support immune function, energy production, bone health, and cardiovascular health.

3. Healthy Fats: Sourced from nuts, seeds, and avocados, healthy fats are essential for brain function, hormone production, and the absorption of fat-soluble vitamins. They also contribute to heart health by improving cholesterol levels.

4. Lean Proteins: Proteins from fish, poultry, beans, and tofu are crucial for muscle repair, enzyme function, and the production of hormones and antibodies.

5. Antioxidants: Found in a variety of fruits and vegetables, antioxidants help protect the body from oxidative stress and inflammation, reducing the risk of chronic diseases.

6. Complex Carbohydrates: Whole grains and legumes provide complex carbohydrates that offer sustained energy and stabilize blood sugar levels, unlike refined carbohydrates that cause rapid spikes and crashes.

Preparing Your Kitchen: Essential Tools and Ingredients

Here's a comprehensive guide to help you get started:

Essential Tools

1. Quality Chef's Knife: A sharp, versatile knife is crucial for chopping vegetables, fruits, and lean proteins efficiently.

2. Cutting Board: Invest in a sturdy cutting board. Consider having separate boards for vegetables and proteins to avoid cross-contamination.

3. Non-Stick Cookware: Non-stick pans and pots reduce the need for cooking oils, aligning with the Pritikin Diet's focus on low-fat cooking.

4. Steamer Basket: Perfect for steaming vegetables, preserving their nutrients and flavor without added fat.

5. Blender or Food Processor: Useful for making smoothies, soups, and sauces from whole, unprocessed ingredients.

6. Measuring Cups and Spoons: Essential for accurate portion control and following recipes precisely.

7. Mixing Bowls: Various sizes for mixing salads, marinating proteins, and preparing batters.

8. Salad Spinner: Helps in thoroughly washing and drying greens, making salad preparation quicker and easier.

9. Baking Sheets: Ideal for roasting vegetables and baking lean proteins.

10. Storage Containers: Invest in airtight containers to store prepped ingredients and leftovers, ensuring freshness and convenience.

Essential Ingredients

Fresh Produce

1. Vegetables: Leafy greens (spinach, kale), cruciferous vegetables (broccoli, cauliflower), root vegetables (carrots, sweet potatoes), bell peppers, cucumbers, tomatoes.

2. Fruits: Berries, apples, oranges, bananas, pears, and seasonal fruits to add variety and essential vitamins.

Whole Grains

1. Brown Rice: A versatile staple for many dishes.

2. Quinoa: A protein-rich grain alternative.

3. Oats: Ideal for breakfast and baking.

4. Whole Grain Bread and Pasta: Choose whole grain options to ensure higher fiber intake.

Lean Proteins

1. Fish: Salmon, trout, and other fatty fish rich in omega-3 fatty acids.

2. Poultry: Skinless chicken breasts and turkey.

3. Legumes: Beans, lentils, and chickpeas for plant-based protein.

4. Tofu and Tempeh: Excellent sources of plant-based protein.

Healthy Fats

1. Avocados: For healthy monounsaturated fats.

2. Nuts and Seeds: Almonds, walnuts, chia seeds, and flaxseeds, in moderation.

3. Olive Oil: Use sparingly for dressings and cooking.

Dairy and Alternatives

1. Low-Fat Dairy: Greek yogurt, cottage cheese, and skim milk.

2. Non-Dairy Milk: Almond, soy, or oat milk, unsweetened varieties.

Spices and Herbs

1. Fresh and Dried Herbs: Basil, cilantro, parsley, oregano, thyme, rosemary.

2. Spices: Turmeric, cumin, paprika, black pepper, cinnamon, and ginger.

3. Garlic and Onions: Fundamental for flavoring dishes.

Other Essentials

1. Low-Sodium Broth: Vegetable or chicken broth for soups and stews.

2. Whole Wheat Flour: For baking and cooking.

3. Natural Sweeteners: Honey or pure maple syrup, used sparingly.

Preparation Tips

1. Meal Planning: Plan your meals for the week, including breakfast, lunch, dinner, and snacks. This helps in making a precise shopping list and avoids impulse buys.

2. Batch Cooking: Prepare large batches of grains, proteins, and chopped vegetables to streamline meal preparation during the week.

3. Portion Control: Use measuring tools to ensure proper portion sizes, helping to avoid overeating and maintain balanced nutrition.

4. Experiment with Recipes: Try new recipes to keep your meals interesting and prevent dietary monotony.

Healthy Black Bean Salad

Prep Time: 20 minutes

Total Time: 20 minutes

Course: Dinner, Entertaining, Leftovers, Lunch, Main Dish, Salad, Side Dish, Snack

Yield: 2 servings

Materials

- 1 cup black beans cooked, no-salt-added
- 1/4 cup red onions diced
- 1/4 cup green bell peppers small diced
- 1/4 cup yellow bell peppers small diced
- 1 teaspoon cumin
- 1 tablespoon cilantro leaves picked and chopped
- 1 tablespoon lime juice
- 1/2 teaspoon black pepper freshly ground

Instructions

• In a medium-sized bowl, mix all ingredients. Let marinate for 2 hours before serving.

Coriander-Crusted Scallops With Curried Cauliflower

Course: Lunch, Main Course, Main Dish, Side Dish

Yield: 6 people

Materials

FOR CORIANDER-CRUSTED SCALLOPS:

• 1 tablespoon coarsely ground coriander

• 1 teaspoon cilantro finely chopped

• 1/4 teaspoon black peppercorns ground

• 1/4 teaspoon porcini powder

• 18 large scallops

• 1/4 cup orange juice

FOR CURRIED CAULIFLOWER:

• 2 heads caulifower chopped

• 2 teaspoons madras curry powder

- 1 leek white only chopped

- 3 cups water

- 1 cup celery root peeled and diced

- 1/2 teaspoon black peppercorns ground

- 2 tablespoons garlic minced

- 1/2 cup milk (skim)

Instructions

FOR CORIANDER-CRUSTED SCALLOPS:

- Mix all spices together. Coat scallops with spice mixture.

- In a very hot nonstick skillet, sear scallops. Do not move scallops for 1 minute.

- Flip scallops and sear for 30 seconds more.

- Add orange juice, and cook for 30 seconds more.

FOR CURRIED CAULIFLOWER

- In a stockpot, bring all ingredients, except the milk, to a boil, and continue boiling until vegetables are very soft, about 45 minutes.

- Add milk, and cook on medium heat until mostly reduced.

- Puree.

• Spoon Curried Cauliflower onto individual dishes. Top with scallops.

Asian Lettuce Wraps

Prep Time: 45 minutes

Active Time: 15 minutes

Total Time: 1 hour

Course: Appetizer, Dinner, Entertaining, Lunch, Main Course, Main Dish, Side Dish, Vegetarian

Yield: 12 servings

Materials

• 8 ounces soba noodles uncooked

• 1 quart water

• 1 teaspoon sesame oil roasted

• 1/4 cup scallions sliced

• 1 tablespoon vinegar rice

• 2 pints cucumbers hothouse, cut into long thin strips

• 1/2 cup lemon juice freshly squeezed

• 1 tablespoon paprika

• 2 carrots cut into long thin strips

- 3 tablespoons cilantro leaves picked from stems and chopped
- 1 teaspoon ginger root freshly grated
- 1/2 cup plain yogurt, fat free
- 3 sprigs dill freshly chopped
- 1 pint bean sprouts (fresh)
- 1 pint alfalfa sprouts (fresh)
- 4 cups red bell peppers cut into long thin strips
- 1 cup rice (basmati brown) cooked
- 2 pounds butterhead lettuce separated into 12 leaves or more

Instructions

- Cook soba noodles in 1 quart of water until soft. Drain. Cool in ice water for about 2 minutes. When cool, remove noodles and toss with sesame oil, scallions, and vinegar. Let sit for 1 hour.
- Meanwhile, mix cucumbers, lemon juice, and paprika. Let marinate for 1 hour.
- Steam carrots (about 2 minutes) and let cool.
- In a blender, mix cilantro, ginger, yogurt, and dill.

• On a large serving plate, serve small piles of the following: 1) noodles, 2) cucumbers, 3) carrots, 4) bean sprouts, 5) alfalfa sprouts, 5) red bell peppers, 6) rice, and 7) whole lettuce leaves.

• Accompany with yogurt sauce.

• Spoon into each lettuce leaf desired ingredients, including sauce, and wrap.

Italian White Bean & Spinach Stew

Course: Lunch, Side Dish, Soup, Soup/Stew, Vegetarian

Yield: 20 people (8 oz portions)

Materials
• 1/4 quart white wine
• 1/2 qts red onion finely diced
• 1/4 cup garlic chopped
• 1/2 qts red bell pepper sliced
• 15 tomatoes Roma (fresh & seeded) finely chopped
• 1 quart white beans cooked
• 1/4 cup balsamic vinegar
• 1/4 cup soy sauce (lite)

- 1/4 cup black pepper
- 1/2 cup basil (fresh) chopped
- 3 pounds spinach fresh picked & sliced

Instructions

- Cook the onion, garlic and red pepper in white wine for about 10 minutes.
- Add the tomato and white beans.
- Mix well and cook for another 20 minutes, stirring occasionally.
- Add spinach.
- Serve hot

Pritikin Caesar Salad

Prep Time: 20 minutes

Total Time: 20 minutes

Course: Lunch, Salad

Yield: 2 people

Materials

- 1 box tofu (lite silken)

- 1/4 cup lemon juice

- 3/4 tablespoon Angostura Worcestershire sauce

- 2 tablespoons Dijon mustard, no-salt-added

- 2 cups white balsamic vinegar

- 2 tablespoons garlic minced

- 1 tablespoon 100% apple juice concentrate (found in freezer sections) thawed, undiluted

- 2 ounces water

- 4 cups chopped Romaine lettuce

- 1 teaspoon Parmesan cheese fat-free

Instructions

- In a food processor or blender, combine all ingredients except Romaine and Parmesan.
- Process until dressing is completely smooth and creamy.
- Combine desired amount of dressing with Romaine and Parmesan.
- Refrigerate remaining dressing.

Dal

Prep Time: 15 minutes

Active Time: 40 minutes

Total Time: 55 minutes

Course: Main Course, Soup

Cuisine: Easy, Indian, Vegan, Vegetarian

Yield: 6 cups

Materials

• 1.5 cups lentils (dried) rinsed and drained

• 5 cups vegetable stock low sodium

• 1 tablespoon red chili pepper flakes

• 1/2 tablespoon turmeric ground

• 1.5 cups onions chopped

• 3 garlic cloves minced

• 1 tablespoon fresh ginger peeled and minced

• 1 tablespoon cumin ground

• 1/2 tablespoon curry powder

• Fresh lemon juice to taste

Instructions

• In a large stockpot, combine lentils, 4 cups of stock, red pepper flakes, and turmeric.

• Bring to a boil, then reduce to simmer.

• Stir occasionally and cook until lentils are just tender, about 25 minutes.

• Add more liquid, if necessary, to prevent sticking.

• While lentils are cooking, heat a large nonstick saute pan to medium high. Saute onions, garlic, ginger, cumin, and curry until onions start soften, about 5 minutes.

• If the mixture is sticking and browning too quickly, pour in a small amount of stock and scrape the bottom of pan to release any bits of food that are sticking.

• Stir in cooked lentils and more stock, to desired consistency.

• Simmer for 10 minutes. Add lemon juice.

Notes

1. Dal is delicious served over brown basmati rice, regular brown rice, or with whole-wheat pita bread and raita, an Indian side dish of yogurt, cucumber, and seasonings.

Thai-Style Vegetable Stir Fry

Prep Time: 30 minutes

Active Time: 10 minutes

Total Time: 40 minutes

Course: Dinner, Entertaining, Vegetarian

Yield: 4 people

Materials

• 1 tablespoon garlic chopped

• 1 tablespoon ginger root peeled and chopped

• 1/4 cup 100% frozen apple juice concentrate thawed, undiluted

• 2 tablespoons Dijon mustard, no-salt-added

• 1/4 cup vegetable stock (low-sodium)

• 1 zucchini sliced into thin strips

• 1 red bell pepper sliced into thin strips

• 1 Vidalia onion sliced into thin strips

• 1 head broccoli stems and florets chopped

• 1/2 pound button mushrooms wiped clean, sliced in half

• 1/4 bunch cilantro leaves chopped

• 2 tablespoons cornstarch

• 2 tablespoons water

Instructions

• In a wok or nonstick skillet, sauté garlic and ginger until glossy.

• Add apple juice, mustard, and half of vegetable stock, stirring to combine.

• Add remaining ingredients (except cornstarch and water). Sauté for 5 minutes.

• Whisk cornstarch in water, and add to thicken stir fry.

Fish en Papillote

Course: Lunch, Main Course, Main Dish

Yield: 4 people

Materials

• Parchment paper

• Four 4-ounce servings of seafood

• 2 tomatoes chopped

• 1 tablespoon fresh thyme leaves

• 1 red onion chopped

• 2 tablespoon fresh dill chopped

• 1/4 teaspoon black peppercorns ground

• 1/2 cup white wine

Instructions

• Preheat oven to 400°F.

• Cut four large rectangles of parchment paper and fold in half; unfold. Set aside.

• Marinate the fish in remaining ingredients. Place fish in parchment paper, and top with the vegetables and herbs from the marinade. Fold top half of parchment paper over fish and crimp to seal. Place on two baking sheets. Bake until done, about 10 minutes. Open the top of each paper and serve immediately.

Israeli Salad

Course: Lunch, Salad, Side Dish, Vegetarian
Cuisine: Mediterranean, Middle Eastern, Vegan, Vegetarian
Yield: 4 people

Materials

• 1 cup cucumber peeled & diced

• 1 cup tomato diced

- 2 tablespoon parseley picked & chopped

- 1/4 teaspoon black peppercorns ground

- 1 teaspoon coriander

- 1 teaspoon oregano

- 1 teaspoon papaya (fresh)

- 1/4 cup garlic Place garlic cloves on a nonstick sheet in the oven and bake at 350 degrees for 12 to 15 minutes on one side, then 5 minutes on the other, till brown.

- 1/2 cup red pepper diced

- 4 lemon juiced

Instructions

- Mix all ingredients together and let sit 15 minutes in the refrigerator before serving.

Potato Kugel

Course: Appetizer, Lunch, Vegetarian

Cuisine: American, Continental, International, Vegetarian

Yield: 12 people

Materials

- 12 potatoes (for baking) peeled

- 3 onions peeled

- 3 tablespoons garlic chopped

- 1 cup egg beaters

- 1 tablespoons black peppercorns ground

- 1 tablespoon paprika

- 1 cup potato starch

Instructions

- Shred potato & onions.

- In a colander let potato drain for 5 minutes.

- Press to release more water and drain for 3 minutes more.

- In a large bowl whisk together eggbeaters, garlic, pepper, paprika.

- Whip until well combined.

- Whip in potato starch until fluffy.

- Add potato and onion.

- Put into baking pan about 1 ½ inches thick.

- Cook covered at 350 degrees for 45 minutes, uncover and cook for 10 minutes more until light brown.

- Let sit for 5 minutes before cutting.

Breakfast Quesadilla

Course: Appetizer, Breakfast, Lunch, Vegetarian

Cuisine: American, Mexican, Vegetarian

Yield: 2 people

Materials

• 1 thin bread whole wheat

• 3 tablespoons shredded mozzarella (fat free)

• 1 cup vegetables (assorted) diced

• 1/2 cup egg whites

• 1/4 teaspoon black pepper ground

• 1 tablespoon cilantro (optional) chopped

• 2 tablespoons sour cream, fat free

• 1/4 cup pico de gallo or no salt added Enrico's salsa

Instructions

• In a skillet sauté vegetable until begin to brown; add egg whites and scramble season with black pepper.

• On a warm griddle or flat top grill place thin bread and warm on one side.

• Turn bread on the other side and spread cheese all over the bread.

• Spread cooked vegetables egg mixture on half of the bread only.

• When cheese begins to melt, fold in half to cover the vegetable scramble. Use a lifter to press firmly. Flip on the other side for 2 minutes and press.

• Cut into four pieces and serve two pieces per person with fat free sour cream and Pico de Gallo.

Moroccan Vegetable Stew

Course: Soup/Stew, Vegetarian

Cuisine: African, Mediterranean, Vegan, Vegetarian Yield: 6 people

Materials

• 1/2 cup onion peeled & diced

• 1/2 cup carrots peeled & sliced

• 1/2 cup eggplant peeled & diced

• 1/2 cup red pepper julienne

• 1/2 cup tomato diced

• 1 cup garbanzo beans soaked & rinsed

• 1/2 teaspoon paprika

• 2 tablespoon raisins

• 1 tablespoon parsley picked & chopped

• 1/4 teaspoon crushed red pepper

• 1/4 cup garlic chopped

• 1 tablespoon toasted cariander seeds, ground

• 1 tablespoon cumin seed toasted & ground

• 1/2 cup butternut squash

Instructions

• In a hot stockpot cook eggplant, squash, tomato, onion, & raisins.

• Cook for 30 minutes and add remaining ingredients (except parsley).

• Cook for 20 minutes more.

• When all vegetables are cooked add parsley & serve immediately.

Marinated Italian Vegetables

Course: Appetizer, Lunch, Salad, Vegetarian

Yield: 20 people

Materials

- 2 heads broccoli cut into florets
- 5 heads cauliflower cut into florets
- 1 pound mushrooms halved
- 3 red bell peppers julienne (cut into long strips)
- 1 pound green peas
- 8 carrots sliced

DRESSING

- 1 red onion
- 1 red bell pepper
- 1 green bell pepper
- 1 yellow bell pepper
- 4 cups white balsamic vinegar
- 1 cup Dijon mustard (low-sodium)
- 1/4 cup Italian herbs (a blend)

Instructions

- Cut vegetables (broccoli through carrots) as described.
- Blanch or steam vegetables until tender, but not fully cooked.

• Place vegetables in refrigerator to cool.

• For dressing, place vegetables (onion and peppers) in food processor and process until liquefied.

• Add vinegar, mustard, and herbs. Process until well mixed.

• Place vegetables in a bowl and toss with dressing.

• Refrigerate until chilled.

Couscous

Course: Salad, Side Dish, Vegetarian

Cuisine: International, Vegetarian

Yield: 6 people

Materials

• 12 ounces cous cous

• 15 ounces water

• 1 teaspoon granulated garlic

• 1/2 teaspoon oregano

• 1/4 teaspoon black peppercorns ground

Instructions

• Boil water with spices

• When fully boiling pour over cous cous

• Cover and let sit for 8 minutes

• Fluff with a fork

Notes

1. Make your own all-purpose seasoning by blending ingredients such as paprika, garlic powder, onion powder, dried oregano, and dried basil. You can also purchase our chefs' Pritikin All-Purpose Season Seasoning in the Online Store

Pasta Primavera In Roasted Garlic & Caramelized Onion Sauce

Course: Dinner, Lunch, Main Course, Main Dish, Vegetarian

Cuisine: American, Italian, Vegan, Vegetarian

Yield: 6 6-ounce per serving

Materials

• 1 cup carrots julienned (cut into long thin strips)

• 1 cup zucchini julienned

• 1 cup yellow squash julienned

• 1 cup domestic mushrooms sliced

• 1 red onion julienned

• 1/4 cup fresh garlic chopped

• 1 cup asparagus sliced

• 1 cup arugula leaves chiffonade (stack leaves and roll tightly, then cut across with a sharp knife to produce fine ribbons)

• 1/8 cup basil leaves chiffonaide

• 1/8 cup Italian parsley chopped

• 2 cups Roasted Garlic & Caramelized Onion Sauce

• Italian Seasoning (salt-free) to taste

• black pepper to taste

• 2 pounds pasta (whole-wheat) cooked

Instructions

• In large hot nonstick skillet, sauté carrots, zucchini, squash, mushrooms, and onions till slightly browned, about 2 minutes. Add garlic. Sauté 30 seconds.

• Add asparagus. Continue sautéing till asparagus is tender. (Time depends on thickness of asparagus.)

• Add arugula, basil, parsley, roasted garlic/onion sauce, salt-free Italian seasoning, and black pepper. Heat.

• When heated, add just-cooked pasta. Toss and serve.

Vegetable Sushi

Course: Appetizer, Dinner, Entertaining, Lunch, Main Course, Main Dish, Side Dish, Vegetarian

Cuisine: Asian, Vegan, Vegetarian

Yield: 4 people

Materials

• 1 cup brown rice, short grain dry

• 1.5 cup water

• 2 tablespoons rice vinegar

• 1 teaspoon Splenda

• 1/2 teaspoon ginger minced

• 2 cups cucumber peeled and sliced

• 4 ounce red pepper sliced

- 1 carrot julienned, steamed, and iced

- 1 ounce wasabi paste

- 1 ounce scallion

- 4 spears asparagus steamed and iced

- 4 nori sheets

- 1 ounce ginger picked

Instructions

- Soak rice in cold water for 20 minutes. Drain

- In a stockpot bring to boil 1 ½ cups water, Splenda, vinegar and ½ teaspoon ginger

- When water is boiling add rice. Lower heat and cover

- Cook until rice is soft on low heat, about 35 minutes. Let rice cool

- Lay out Nori and place rice on top, leaving 1/3 of Nori uncovered

- Lay in cucumber, carrot, asparagus, red pepper, scallion and pickled ginger

- Roll tight

- Serve with rice vinegar and Wasabi paste

Red Pepper Gumbo

Course: Soup/Stew, Vegetarian

Cuisine: American, International, Vegan, Vegetarian Yield: 10 people

Materials

• 2 red peppers

• 2 green peppers

• 2 yellow peppers

• 1/2 head fennel diced

• 1 leek sliced

• 1/2 cup garlic chopped

• 1 cup okra fresh sliced

• 1/2 chipotle pepper de-seeded & diced

• 1 carrot diced

• 3 q stalks celery diced

• 2 tablespoons thyme picked & chopped

• 3 quart vegetable stock

• 1 pint tomato puree (low sodium)

• 1 teaspoon gumbo file

• 1 teaspoon coriander ground

• 1 teaspoon soy sauce, low sodium

- 1.5 teaspoon black peppercorns ground

- 1/4 cup cornstarch

- 1/4 cup cold water

Instructions

- Roast Peppers, peel & de-seed. Then diced.

- Brown all vegetables in a large hot stockpot.

- Deglaze with tomato sauce and stock.

- Add seasonings, bring to boil and cook for 1-½ hours at a simmer.

- Thicken with cornstarch & water mixture.

- Serve hot.

Vegetarian Chili

Prep Time: 30 minutes

Active Time: 1 hour 10 minutes

Total Time: 1 hour 40 minutes

Course: Lunch, Main Dish, Side Dish, Soup/Stew, Vegetarian

Cuisine: American, Comfort Food, International, Vegetarian

Yield: 12 half-cup servings

Materials

- 1 cup red bell pepper diced
- 1 cup poblano pepper diced
- 1 cup cubanelle pepper diced
- 1 cup So Soya (TVP) ground. See Recipe notes.
- 1 cup red onion diced
- 1/4 cup garlic chopped
- 3 tb green grotto
- 2 cup corn kernels (fresh or frozen)
- 3 cups red beans cooked, (If using canned varieties, purchase no-salt-added)
- 2 tsp oregano dry
- 1 tsp basil chopped
- 2 tsp coriander
- 1 tsp chipotle chili powder
- 1 tsp paprika
- 1 tsp Southwest seasoning
- 1/3 bottle Enrico mild salsa
- 1 tb balsamic glaze
- 1 cup tomato puree no-salt-added

- 1/2 cup unsweetened ketchup

- 1 quart vegetable stock (low-sodium)

- 1/4 tsp liquid smoke

- 2 tb fresh cilantro, chopped added at the end

- 2 tb fresh parsley, chopped added at the end.

Instructions

- In a large nonstick stockpot, sauté bell peppers, onion, and garlic at medium-high heat until brown, about 3 minutes.

- Meanwhile, soak So Soya in ½ cup hot water for about 5 minutes. Drain excess liquid. Add So-Soya and All Purpose Seasoning to stockpot, and cook for 3 minutes. Add remaining ingredients, except cilantro and parsley, and simmer for 1 hour.

- Finish off with freshly chopped cilantro.

- Serve with whole-wheat, low-sodium pita chips, brown rice, mashed potatoes, or simply by itself.

Notes

1. So Soya is a dehydrated soybean product. It is available in some supermarkets nationwide as well.

2. Make your own All Purpose Seasoning by blending granulated onion, granulated garlic, salt-free lemon pepper, and paprika.

3. Veggie Grated Topping, Parmesan, is made by Galaxy Nutritional Foods. It's in grocery stores. Don't go overboard on it because it does have added sodium.

Red Pepper Gumbo

Course: Soup/Stew, Vegetarian
Cuisine: American, International, Vegan, Vegetarian Yield: 10 people

Materials
• 2 red peppers
• 2 green peppers
• 2 yellow peppers
• 1/2 head fennel diced
• 1 leek sliced
• 1/2 cup garlic chopped
• 1 cup okra fresh sliced
• 1/2 chipotle pepper de-seeded & diced

- 1 carrot diced

- 3 q stalks celery diced

- 2 tablespoons thyme picked & chopped

- 3 quart vegetable stock

- 1 pint tomato puree (low sodium)

- 1 teaspoon gumbo file

- 1 teaspoon coriander ground

- 1 teaspoon soy sauce, low sodium

- 1.5 teaspoon black peppercorns ground

- 1/4 cup cornstarch

- 1/4 cup cold water

Instructions

- Roast Peppers, peel & de-seed. Then diced.

- Brown all vegetables in a large hot stockpot.

- Deglaze with tomato sauce and stock.

- Add seasonings, bring to boil and cook for 1-½ hours at a simmer.

- Thicken with cornstarch & water mixture.

- Serve hot.

Vegetarian Chili

Slow but oh-so-good cooking. That's what this vegetarian chili's all about. Want to add leftover shredded roasted chicken or turkey breast. Go right ahead. Poultry- or veggie-style, it's a wonderful one-pot dish.

Prep Time: 30 minutes
Active Time: 1 hour 10 minutes
Total Time: 1 hour 40 minutes
Course: Lunch, Main Dish, Side Dish, Soup/Stew, Vegetarian
Cuisine: American, Comfort Food, International, Vegetarian
Yield: 12 half-cup servings

Materials
• 1 cup red bell pepper diced
• 1 cup poblano pepper diced
• 1 cup cubanelle pepper diced
• 1 cup So Soya (TVP) ground.
• 1 cup red onion diced
• 1/4 cup garlic chopped

• 3 tb green grotto

• 2 cup corn kernels (fresh or frozen)

• 3 cups red beans cooked, (If using canned varieties, purchase no-salt-added)

• 2 tsp oregano dry

• 1 tsp basil chopped

• 2 tsp coriander

• 1 tsp chipotle chili powder

• 1 tsp paprika

• 1 tsp Southwest seasoning

• 1/3 bottle Enrico mild salsa

• 1 tb balsamic glaze

• 1 cup tomato puree no-salt-added

• 1/2 cup unsweetened ketchup

• 1 quart vegetable stock (low-sodium)

• 1/4 tsp liquid smoke

• 2 tb fresh cilantro, chopped added at the end

• 2 tb fresh parsley, chopped added at the end

Instructions

• In a large nonstick stockpot, sauté bell peppers, onion, and garlic at medium-high heat until brown, about 3 minutes.

• Meanwhile, soak So Soya in ½ cup hot water for about 5 minutes. Drain excess liquid. Add So-Soya and All Purpose Seasoning to stockpot, and cook for 3 minutes.

• Add remaining ingredients, except cilantro and parsley, and simmer for 1 hour.

• Finish off with freshly chopped cilantro.

• Serve with whole-wheat, low-sodium pita chips, brown rice, mashed potatoes, or simply by itself.

Notes

1. So Soya is a dehydrated soybean product. It is available in some supermarkets nationwide as well.

2. Make your own All Purpose Seasoning by blending granulated onion, granulated garlic, salt-free lemon pepper, and paprika.

3. Veggie Grated Topping, Parmesan, is made by Galaxy Nutritional Foods. It's in grocery stores. Don't go overboard on it because it does have added sodium.

Moroccan Lentil Soup

Course: Appetizer, Soup, Vegetarian

Cuisine: Mediterranean, Middle Eastern, Vegan, Vegetarian

Yield: 16 people

Materials

• 2 onions chopped

• 4 cloves fresh garlic minced

• 4 stalks celery sliced

• 1/2 teaspoon salt

• 1 teaspoon black peppercorns ground

• 1 teaspoon turmeric

• 1 teaspoon cumin

• 1/4 teaspoon ground cinnamon

• 1 pinch saffron

• 1 bay leaf

• 2 tablespoon tomato puree

• 2 potato peeled & diced

• 1 pound red lentils

• 2 quarts vegetable stock (water or low-sodium)

• 6 plum tomato diced

• 1/2 bunch cilantro chopped

Instructions

• Saute onions & garlic until light brown.

• Add celery and cook 3 minutes, until soft.

• Add salt, pepper, tumeric, cumin, ginger, cinnamon, saffron, bay leaf and cook for half an hour over low heat.

• Add tomato puree, potato, lentil, water & cook for 45 minutes.

• Add diced tomato and cook for 5 minutes.

• Garnish with cilantro.

PRITIKIN STYLE MALAYSIAN CHICKEN

Ready In: 1hr 25mins

Ingredients: 18

Serves: 6

INGREDIENTS

• 48 ounces chicken breast halves, skinned

• 1 cup chicken stock or 1 cup vegetable stock, minus fat

- 1 cup tomato sauce

- 1/2 red wine vinegar

- 2 tablespoons red Burgundy wine

- 2 tablespoons frozen apple juice concentrate

- 2 teaspoons soy sauce

- 1 lemon, juice of

- 2 garlic cloves

- 2 teaspoons curry powder

- 2 teaspoons powdered ginger

- 2 teaspoons cardamom

- 1 teaspoon ground cumin

- 1 teaspoon onion powder

- 1/2 teaspoon garlic powder

- 1/2 teaspoon red pepper flakes

- 1/2 teaspoon dry mustard

- 1 cup nonfat yogurt

DIRECTIONS

1. Place chicken pieces in a large bowl or pan. Place all the remaining ingredients, except yogurt, in a blender, and blend.

2. Pour the

3. Mixture over the chicken, turning to coat well. Cover and marinate over night in the refrigerator.

4. About 1 hour before serving, transfer chicken and marinade to a baking dish. Cover and bake at 350 degrees for 50 minutes, or until chicken is nearly done.

5. Remove from oven and spoon some of the chicken sauce into a small bowl. Allow sauce to cool slightly, then add the yogurt to the bowl and mix with the sauce.

6. Pour mixture over the chicken. Cover and return to the oven for 20 minutes, or until the chicken is tender.

7. The sauce may curdle slightly, but this will not affect the taste or quality of the dish.

8. Garnish with orange slices and parsley.

9. You can also sprinkle 1 1/2 cups of cooked peas over the chicken breast just before serving.

Lebanese Lentil Soup

Prep Time: 25 minutes

Active Time: 45 minutes

Total Time: 1 hour 10 minutes

Course: Leftovers, Snack, Soup

Cuisine: Easy, Middle Eastern, Vegetarian

Yield: 10 1-cup servings

Materials

- 1 cup lentils dry
- 1 quart vegetable broth low-sodium
- 1 cup onions chopped
- 1/2 cup celery chopped
- 1/2 cup red bell peppers diced
- 1 cup carrots chopped
- 1/2 cup fresh garlic minced
- 1/2 tbsp oregano leaves dry
- 1/2 tbsp soy sauce, low sodium
- 1/2 tbsp black pepper freshly ground
- 1/2 cup fresh basil leaves chopped
- 1/2 teaspoon fresh thyme leaves chopped
- 1 pint RW Knudsen Very Veggie Juice (Low Sodium)

Instructions

• Wash lentils. In a large stockpot, combine lentils and all ingredients except basil, thyme, and vegetable juice. Bring to a boil.

• Reduce heat and simmer, covered, for 30 minutes, stirring occasionally.

• Add remaining ingredients, adjust seasonings as desired, and simmer 15 more minutes.

Notes

1. To wash lentils thoroughly, place them in a large bowl and fill it with cold water. Scoop up handfuls of the lentils and scrub them by rubbing your palms together. The water will likely turn a little dirty. Drain the water and refill with clean water. Swish lentils in water and drain. Repeat until the water runs clear.

Thai Coleslaw

Course: Lunch, Side Dish

Cuisine: Asian, Vegan, Vegetarian

Yield: 5 people

Materials

SALAD

• 1.5 cup green cabbage shredded

• 1.5 cup red cabbage shredded

• 1 cup carrot shredded & rinsed

DRESSING

• 1/2 cup brown rice vinegar

• 1 tablespoon apple juice concentrate

• 1 tablespoon basil chiffonaide

• 1/4 cup ginger minced

• 2 teaspoon garlic minced

• 1 teaspoon dill minced

• 1 teaspoon tarragon minced

• 1 teaspoon Dijon mustard

Instructions

• Mix dressing in a cuisenart.

• Combine with vegetables and let chill for one hour.

Notes

1. Serving Size: 4 ounces

Grilled Ratatouille

Prep Time: 15 minutes

Active Time: 10 minutes

Total Time: 25 minutes

Course: Lunch, Main Course, Main Dish, Vegetarian

Cuisine: American, French, Fusion, International, Vegan, Vegetarian

Yield: 12 people

Materials

- 1 pound shiitake mushrooms reconstituted in hot water
- 4 large zucchini thickly sliced
- 3 yellow squash thickly sliced
- 2 red onion thickly sliced
- 3 japanese eggplant thickly sliced
- Oregano, red wine vinegar, and ground celery seeds to taste

Instructions

- Season vegetables with black pepper, freshly chopped rosemary, dry oregano, red wine vinegar, and ground celery seeds

- Grill and lay out to cool
- When cool, dice all vegetables and serve

Spanish-Style Omelet

Course: Breakfast, Lunch, Main Course, Main Dish, Vegetarian

Cuisine: Vegetarian

Materials

- Olive oil cooking spray
- 1/2 cup onion chopped
- 2 cloves garlic minced
- 2 medium potatoes (for baking) washed and diced small
- 1 green pepper diced
- 1 ripe tomato diced
- 1 teaspoon oregano (dry)
- 1 teaspoon rosemary (dry) chopped
- Coarse ground black pepper to taste
- 1.5 cups egg substitute (nonfat)

Instructions

• Generously spray a large nonstick skillet with olive oil cooking spray and heat over medium-high heat.

• Sauté the onion and garlic until golden, about 2 minutes.

• Add the potatoes, green pepper, tomato, and seasonings.

• Cook until tender, stirring frequently, about 5 to 6 minutes.

• Transfer potato mixture to a plate.

• Clean and dry the skillet.

• Spray again with olive oil cooking spray and place over medium-high heat.

• Allow the pan to get hot, then pour the egg sub-stitute into the pan.

• Using a rubber spatula, fold the egg from the outside into the center until the eggs are almost set.

• Add the potato mixture on top; allow all to heat through, keeping the omelet loose from the pan with the spatula.

• Remove from the stove.

• Cut into quarters and serve.

Zucchini & Garbanzo Salad

Course: Appetizer, Salad, Vegetarian

Cuisine: American, International, Vegan, Vegetarian Yield:
12 people

Materials

- 2 zucchini julienned (cut into long thin strips)
- 2 yellow squash julienned
- 1 red onion julienned
- 1 red pepper, julienned
- 1 carrot peeled and julienned
- 4 lemons juiced
- 1/2 bunch dill chopped
- 1 tablespoon coriander
- 1 tablespoon paprika
- 1/4 teaspoon black peppercons ground
- 1/2 cup water
- 6 ounces garbanzo beans cooked and cooled

Instructions

- Mix zucchini, squash, onion, lemon juice, dill, coriander, paprika, pepper, and water together.

- Let marinate for 1 hour.
- Sprinkle each salad with one-half ounce of beans.

Moroccan Poached Fish

Course: Dinner, Lunch, Main Course, Main Dish
Cuisine: Fish, Mediterranean, Middle Eastern
Yield: 4 people

Materials

- 16 ounces fish cut into 4-ounce portions.
- 6 large red tomatoes shredded
- 1/4 cup fresh garlic minced
- 1 jalapeno pepper finely chopped, seedes removed
- 1/2 bunch cilantro leaves chopped
- 1/2 bunch Italian parsley leaves chopped
- 1 tablespoon coriander seeds toasted and ground
- 1/2 tablespoon cumin seeds toasted and ground
- 1/4 teaspoon black pepper freshly ground
- 2 lemons juiced

Instructions

• In a large hot nonstick skillet, cook shredded tomatoes over medium heat until they are reduced by half.

• In a food processor, puree the rest of the ingredients, except lemon juice.

• When tomatoes are reduced, add the pureed mixture to skillet.

• Bring to a complete boil, and mix well.

• Cool, then add lemon juice.

• Preheat oven to 350 degrees F.

• In a baking pan, lay out fish, all in one layer.

• Pour skillet mixture over fish.

• Cover with foil and bake in oven until fish is cooked, about 20 minutes.

• Serve.

Notes

1. To toast seeds, place them over high heat on the stove in a small heavy skillet. Toss them frequently until fragrant, about 2 to 4 minutes.

Potato Latke

Course: Appetizer, Entertaining, Lunch

Cuisine: American, Easy, International, Vegetarian Yield: 12 people

Materials

• 6 Idaho potato, peeled & steamed

• 1 onion peeled

• 1/4 teaspoon black peppercorns ground

• 2 egg whites

• 2 tablespoons potato starch

Instructions

• Grate steamed potato on a box grater.

• Grate onion on a box grater.

• In a large bowl whip egg whites with pepper & potato starch. Fold in Onions & potato.

• Bake at 350 degrees until light brown or saute in a hot skillet with spray until brown. Serve immediately

Tandoori Tofu

Course: Appetizer, Dinner, Lunch, Main Dish, Vegetarian

Cuisine: American, International, Vegetarian

Yield: 4 people

Materials

- 2 teaspoon cumin seed

- 3 cloves

- 3 ounces yogurt fat free

- 3 tablespoons garlic chopped

- 3 tablespoon ginger chopped

- 1.25 tablespoon chilli power

- 1.25 tablespoon paprika

- 1 tablespoon soy sauce, low sodium

- 16 oz firm tofu cut into 4 oz portions

- 2 cups yogurt fat free

- 1 red onion julienne

- 1 cucumber peeled, de-seeded & grated

- 1 lemon juiced

- 1 tablespoon mint (fresh) chopped

- 1 tablespoon cilantro chopped

Instructions

• TOFU

• Toast and grind cloves & cumin.

• Mix well with remainder of ingredients, except tofu, in Cuisenart.

• Marinate with tofu for 24 hours.

• Grill tofu and serve with cucumber raita

• RAITA

• Line a colander with cheesecloth and put in yogurt.

• Cover and refrigerate overnight.

• Discard liquid and mix all ingredients well with a whisk.

• Serve cold.

Grilled Fish with Baby Kale

Prep Time: 10 minutes

Active Time: 12 minutes

Total Time: 22 minutes

Course: Dinner, Lunch, Main Course, Main Dish

Cuisine: Caribbean, Fish

Yield: 5 people

Materials

• 5 large swai fillets or other mild white fish

• 1 large package kale (baby)

• 2 cloves garlic minced

• 2 limes zest and juiced

• 1 handful cilantro (fresh leaves)

• pepper to taste

• cooking spray oil non-stick

• rice (whole grain) cooked

Instructions

• Preheat your grill. Lay out 5 large pieces of aluminum foil and lightly spray with non-stick cooking spray. Pile on each foil in order: large stack raw baby kale, 1 piece of fish, lightly pepper, sprinkle on a bit of garlic, the lime zest, a small squeeze of lime juice and a sprinkling of cilantro.

• Repeat for all 5 foils.

• Wrap them up tight and place them on your grill.

• Grill approximately 15 minutes, or until the fish is firm, white and flaky. Serve over whole grain rice!

Seafood Medley

This medley of shrimp, scallops and clams is served in a white wine sauce.

Course: Dinner, Lunch, Main Course, Main Dish
Cuisine: American, Continental, Fusion
Yield: 6 people

Materials
- 12 shimp
- 18 sea scallops
- 24 cherry clams
- 1 tablespoon lemon juice
- 1/4 cup parsley
- 1/4 cup chives
- 1 cup white wine
- 1/2 tablespoon paprika
- 1/2 tablespoon Mrs. Dash
- 1/2 tablespoon white pepper
- 2 tablespoon cornstarch
- 1 tablespoon tomato paste

Instructions

• Marinate the seafood in combination of lemon juice, white wine, parsley, chives and paprika for least for 2 hours.

• Reserve marinade while searing scallops in a non-stick pan.

• Steam shrimp and clams. Remove scallops and shrimp from pan; peel and clean shrimp; set aside.

• Steam sea shallots and garlic, add tomato paste and roast briefly.

• Deglase with marinade.

• Liquefy cornstarch with a little water and stir into the boiling sauce to thicken slightly.

• Add remaining ingredients.

• Serve the seafood with the sauce.

Two-Pepper Risotto

Course: Lunch, Main Dish, Vegetarian

Cuisine: American, Italian, Mediterranean, Vegetarian

Yield: 4 people

Materials

• 1 red bell pepper diced

• 1 green bell pepper diced

• 1 tomato diced

• 1/2 onion diced

• 1 teaspoon garlic minced

• 1 cup rice (arborio)

• 5 cups chicken broth (low sodium)

• 1 tablespoon fresh basil (chopped)

• groun black pepper to taste

• 2 tablespoons Parmesan cheese (fat-free)

Instructions

• Preheat broiler and position rack at the top of the oven.

• Spread peppers, tomato, onion, and garlic on a large baking sheet.

• Broil until golden brown, about 15 minutes. Stir occasionally.

• Combine broiled vegetables with rice and 2 cups broth in a large Dutch oven and place over medium-high heat.

• Cover and bring to a boil.

• Stir frequently and continue cooking uncovered. As the broth evaporates, add more in 1-cup increments.

• Cook until the rice is tender and most of the broth is absorbed, about 35 minutes.

• Stir well and add fresh basil, black pepper, to taste, and Parmesan cheese.

• Allow to stand for a few minutes and serve.

Asian Steamed Fish

Real simple. Real delish. Just about any type of fish works. Good choices in terms of sustainability and omega-3 content include wild salmon, mackerel, and Arctic char (farmed).

Course: Lunch, Main Course, Main Dish
Cuisine: Asian
Yield: 12 servings

Materials
• 1/2 cup garlic minced
• 1/2 cup ginger root grated

- 4 stalks lemongrass sliced

- 1 teaspoon soy sauce low-sodium

- 1/4 cup water

- 1/4 cup vinegar rice

- 3 pounds fish cut into 4-ounce portions

Instructions

- In a food processor, puree all ingredients except fish.

- Marinate fish for 1 hour, then steam until cooked. Steam time will depend on the thickness of your fish.

- Serve hot or cold.

Marinated Chicken

Course: Dinner, Lunch, Main Course, Main Dish

Cuisine: American, Poultry

Yield: 4 people

Materials

- 16 oz chicken breast (boneless, skinless)

- 2 limes juiced

- 1/2 chipotle pepper

- 1 tablespoon water

- 1 teaspoon cider vinegar

- 1 teaspoon garlic

- 1 teaspoon onion

- 1 tomatillo

Instructions

- Puree all ingredients, except chicken, well in a blender.

- Marinate chicken for 3 hours.

- Grill or sear in a Vital Nutrition pan. Cover until cooked.

Cajun-Style Red Beans and Rice

Our Cajun-Style Red Beans and Rice takes just a few minutes to assemble but delivers loads of hearty, snappy flavor.

Prep Time: 20 minutes

Active Time: 7 hours

Total Time: 7 hours 20 minutes

Course: Dinner, Main Course, Side Dish

Cuisine: Easy, Mexican, Vegan, Vegetarian

Yield: 6 one-cup servings

Materials

• 2 cups red kidney beans (dried) rinsed

• 1 cup brown rice uncooked

• 1 red onion chopped

• 1 green bell pepper chopped

• 4 stalks celery chopped

• 6 to 8 cloves garlic minced

• 1/2 cup chives finely chopped

• 4 teaspoons Cajun seasoning (salt-free)

• 1 tablespoon paprika (smoked)

• 5 cups water

Instructions

• Add all your ingredients to your crockpot, veggies on top. Cook on LOW for around 7 hours. Cooking times may vary depending on your crockpot.

Quinoa Salad

Course: Appetizer, Dinner, Lunch, Main Course, Main Dish, Salad, Vegetarian

Cuisine: American, International, Vegan, Vegetarian Yield: 12 people

Materials

Quinoa Salad

- 1.5 cup red quinoa cooked
- 1.5 cup white quinoa can substitute millet
- 1 cup cucumber diced
- 1 cup carrots grated
- 1 cup green onions minced
- 1 cup green bell peppers minced
- 1 cup red bell peppers minced
- 1 cup yellow grape tomatoes halved
- 1 cup red grape tomatoes halved
- 1/2 cup Italian parsley minced
- 1/4 cup cup dill minced
- 1/4 cup basil minced

Zesty Italian Dressing

- 1/2 cup white wine vinegar

- 1/4 cup lemon juice

- 1/2 cup apple juice concentrate

- 1 tsp granulated onion

- 1 tsp granulated garlic

- 1 tsp dry basil

- 1 tsp dry parsley

- 1.5 tsp dry oregano

Instructions

Quinoa Salad

- Mix all ingredients and refrigerate.

Zesty Italian Dressing

- Combine all ingredients in blender and run until smooth.

Notes

1. Add xanthan gum to thicken the dressing as necessary.

Heirloom Tomato Gazpacho

Our Heirloom Tomato Gazpacho is refreshing and so simple. Just combine the following ingredients and refrigerate for 20 minutes.

Prep Time: 25 minutes

Total Time: 25 minutes

Course: Lunch, Snack, Soup

Cuisine: Easy, Latin American, Quick, Vegan, Vegetarian

Yield: 4 people

Materials

• 2 heirloom tomatoes small diced, seeds removed

• 2 cups veggie juice (very low-sodium) such as Knudsen's Very Veggie Juice

• 1 teaspoon coriander ground

• 1 teaspoon Italian parsley leaves picked & chopped

• 1/4 cup vidalia onions minced

• 1 teaspoon garlic minced

• 1/2 jalapeno pepper minced

• 1/2 cup cucumber peeled, seeded, minced

• 1/2 red bell pepper seeded, minced

• 2 tablespoons purple basil (optional) If used, slice thinly.

Instructions

• In a large bowl, combine all ingredients except basil.

• Refrigerate for 20 minutes.

• Pour into serving bowls. Sprinkle ribbons of basil on top.

Couscous & Cherry Tomatoes

Here, from Chef Vincenzo Della Polla, is a simple and savory recipe for whole-wheat couscous. Enjoy it for lunch, as a side dish, or as a hearty snack any time of day.

Course: Salad, Side Dish, Vegetarian
Cuisine: International, Vegan, Vegetarian

Materials
• 1/2 red onion chopped

• 1 cup cherry tomatoes halved

• 1 teaspoon garlic powder

• 1/2 teaspoon oregano dried

- 1/4 teaspoon black pepper

- 1 1/2 cups water

- 1 cup couscous (whole wheat)

Instructions

- Lightly mist a medium nonstick saucepan with canola oil spray and pre-heat over medium-high heat.

- Add onions to pan and sauté until softened, about 2 minutes.

- Add tomatoes, garlic, oregano, black pepper, and water to pan, and bring to a boil.

- Lower heat and simmer until tomatoes begin to soften, about 3 to 4 minutes.

- Meanwhile, place couscous in medium mixing bowl.

- Remove tomato mixture from heat and immediately pour over couscous. Cover and let stand 5 to 8 minutes, until couscous is tender and liquid is absorbed. Stir with fork to fluff before serving.

Matzo Balls

Course: Vegetarian

Cuisine: American, Vegetarian

Yield: 24 people

Materials

• 2 cups whole wheat matzo ground fine in a cuisenart

• 1.5 cups eggbeaters

• 1/4 teaspoon black peppercorns ground

• 1/2 teaspoon granulated garlic

• 1/2 teaspoon granulated onion

• 1/2 teaspoon salt

Instructions

• Whip together all ingredients except matzo meal.

• When fluffy whisk I matzo meal let sit for half an hour.

• Boil 3 gallons water in a large pot.

• Mold matzo balls with vegetable spray on hands to eliminate sticking.

• When all balls are rounded drop into boiling water (must be at a full rolling boil or they will not be fluffy).

• Boil for 20 minutes.

• Reduce heat and simmer for 45 minutes.

• If the water is not boiling, or is not lowered to simmer, the matzo balls will not be right.

Matzo Ball Soup

Course: Appetizer, Side Dish, Soup

Cuisine: American

Yield: 8 people

Materials

• 1/4 cup garlic chopped

• 1/2 medium onion dice

• 1 medium carrots dice

• 2 medium stalks celery dice

• 1/2 leeks white only chopped

• 1 teaspoon paprika

• 1 teaspoon oregano, dry

• 1 tablespoon thyme picked & chopped

• 1.5 quart roasted chicken stock de-fatted

• 1 tablespoon fresh dill

• 1 teaspoon parsley chopped

• 8 Prikikin Matza Balls (see recipe)

Instructions

• Sweat all vegetables with paprika, oregano & thyme.

• When onions are translucent add chicken stock.

• Bring to boil, then simmer for 1 hour.

• When ready to serve add matzo balls, dill & parsley.

Pritikin Kale Chips

The next time you're in the mood for a crunchy snack, try this delicious, nutrient-rich recipe for Pritikin Kale Chips. With less sodium, fewer calories and a lot earthier flavor than their prepackaged counterparts, these kale chips will big a hit. This recipe works best with flat-leaf varieties of kale, not the curly kind.

Course: Appetizer, Entertaining, Vegetarian

Cuisine: American, International

Yield: 1 people

Materials

• 12 or more kale leaves (flat-leaf)

• Oil spray, like Pam

• Seasoning of your choice

Instructions

• Preheat oven to 400 degrees F.

• Use scissors to cut kale leaves into chip-form, about three times the size of a normal potato chip.

• Lay the pieces of kale flat on a nonstick baking sheet. Use more than one sheet if necessary, do not overlap kale pieces.

• Lightly mist kale with oil spray.

• Season with fresh ground pepper and any additional no-salt-added seasoning of your choice. Great options include garlic powder or salt-free Cajun seasoning.

• Bake in over for 10 minutes.

• Allow chips to cool before eating.

Hummus

Course: Dip, Vegetarian

Cuisine: Vegan, Vegetarian

Yield: 6 1/4-cup per serving

Materials

• 3 medium garlic cloves

• 1 15-ounce can garbanzo beans (salt-free) drained

• 2 tablespons fresh lemon juice

• 1 tablespoon white wine worcestershire sauce

• 1 teaspoon Dijon mustard

• 1 teaspoon natural rice vinegar

• 1 teaspoon sesame oil

• 1 parsley or cilantro chopped

Instructions

• In an empty food processor, fitted with the steel chopping blade, feed the garlic through the feed tube while the processor is running to chop the garlic.

• Remove the lid and add the rest of the ingredients. Process until smooth. Transfer the mixture to a bowl and chill until ready to serve. Garnish with chopped parsley or cilantro.

• Serve as a spread or dip with raw vegetables, or use as a sandwich spread on whole-wheat bread or pita with sliced tomato, red onion, cucumber, and lettuce.

PRITIKIN DIET STYLE STIR-FRIED STEAK AND GREEN PEPPERS

Ready In: 1hr

Ingredients: 9

Serves: 4-5

INGREDIENTS

• 1 lb flank steak, trimmed of all visible fat

• 2 tablespoons cornstarch

• 1 tablespoon powdered ginger

• 2 tablespoons frozen apple juice concentrate

• 2 tablespoons soy sauce or 2 tablespoons tamari

• 1/4 cup dry sherry or 1/4 cup wine vinegar

• 3/4 cup stock, without fat

• 4 large green peppers, cut into thin strips

• 1 large carrot, thinly sliced on the diagonal

DIRECTIONS

1. Place flank steak in the freezer until partially frozen. Slice diagonally into very thin strips, cutting across the grain.

2. In a mixing bowl, combine the cornstarch, ginger, apple juice concentrate, soy sauce, sherry, and 1/4 cup of stock.

3. Marinate the meat strips in the mixture for at least 30 minutes, stirring occasionally.(the longer, the better).

4. In a large skillet or wok, heat the remaining stock over high heat. Add the vegetables and stir-fry quickly, no more than 2-3 minutes.

5. Push the vegetables to the sides of the pan, leaving the center empty.

6. Remove the meat from the marinade and stir-fry quickly.

7. Add any remaining marinade, stir until thickened, and then stir in the vegetables.

Chick Pea & Vegetable Curry

Course: Lunch, Side Dish

Cuisine: Vegetarian

Yield: 4 portions

Materials

• 1 medium yellow onion medium dice

• 3 cloves garlic finely chopped

• 3 tablespoon ginger (fresh) finely chopped

• 1/4 cup water

• 1 heaping tablespoon curry powder (madras style)

• 1 heaping teaspoon garam masala

• 1 cup vegetable stock (no salt added)

• 1 can tomatoes (1.5 cup) chopped

• 1.5 cups soy milk (plain)

• 2 cans garbanzo beans (no salt added) drained

• 1 medium bunch collard greens or kale (organic) cut in half horizontally and chopped into ½ inch strips

• 1-2 teaspoons red wine vinegar or apple cider vinegar

Instructions

• Heat a medium sauce pot over medium heat.

• Add the onions, garlic, ginger and water and cook until beginning to soften; about 3-4 minutes. Allow the water to evaporate.

• Add the curry powder, garam masala and sauté for another few minutes to bring out the flavors of the spices, stirring frequently.

• Add the veggie stock, tomatoes, soy milk and garbanzo beans.

• Cook on medium-low heat for about 20 minutes to blend the flavors; reducing the liquid by half.

• Add the collards and vinegar and cook for another 8-10 minutes.

• Taste and adjust seasoning with pepper. Serve on its own or over brown rice.

Notes

1. This recipe is very versatile and goes well with many vegetables. Experiment by adding carrots, broccoli, cauliflower, zucchini or anything else that is in season. Carrots will take a bit longer to cook but you can add the other vegetables at the end and cook for just a few minutes. Frozen peas will also work really well.

Stuffed Japanese Eggplant

Course: Appetizer, Dinner, Lunch, Main Course, Main Dish, Vegetarian

Cuisine: American, Asian, International, Vegan, Vegetarian

Yield: 12 people

Materials

- 12 japanese eggplant halved the long way & scooped
- 1 cup garlic roasted
- 2 pints onions peeled pearl
- 8 cups red Swiss chard sliced thin
- 1 cup seiten fine chopped
- 2 cup corn kernels roasted
- 1 cup beet juice
- 3 sprins rosemary picked & chopped
- 1 bay leaf ground
- 1 cup bread crumbs (whole-wheat)
- 1/4 cup parsley chopped
- 4 limes juiced
- 2 cups pico de gallo

Instructions

• In large hot skillet, sauté the scooped meat from the eggplant, garlic, seiten, onions (whole) & corn.

• Cook for 5 minutes over high heat.

• Reduce temperature and add rosemary, beet juice, Swiss chard, bay leaf & black pepper.

• Cook until mostly dry.

• Take off stove and place mixture in a large bowl.

• Add bread crumbs, parsley & lime juice.

• Stuff into eggplant hold for service.

• Bake eggplant for 30 minutes at 350 degrees.

• Serve immediately. Serve 2 halves with rosemary polenta & warm pico de gallo as sauce.

Hungarian Seiten Stew

Course: Soup/Stew

Cuisine: Asian, Vegetarian

Yield: 12 people

Materials

• 2 pounds seitan

• 2 teaspoon paprika

- 1 teaspoon garlic chopped
- 1 cup onions (vidalia) diced
- 1 teaspoon ginger minced
- 1 teaspoon chili powder
- 8 ounces knudsen very veggie juice
- 1 cup vegetable stock
- 2 pounds potato peeled & diced
- 2 each carrot peeled & diced
- 2 tablespoons fresh thyme picked & chopped
- 1 cup green pepper diced
- 1 each red peppers diced
- 1 each yellow pepper diced
- 1 tablespoon corn starch

Instructions

- In a hot stock pot brown seitan, carrot, onion, garlic & peppers.
- When browned add remaining ingredients and cook for 45 minutes over low heat.
- Serve hot

Pritikin All-Purpose Seasoning

Course: Vegetarian

Cuisine: Vegetarian

Yield: 4 Tablespoons

Materials

• 1 tablespoon granulated onion

• 1 tablespoon granulated garlic

• 1 tablespoon lemon pepper (salt-free)

• 1 tablespoon paprika

Instructions

• Combine all ingredients

Paella

Course: Dinner, Lunch, Main Course, Main Dish, Soup/Stew

Cuisine: Continental, Fish

Yield: 8 14 oz portions

Materials

• 2 cups rice (long gran brown)

- 2 cups fish stock

- 1/2 teaspoon saffron spice

- 1/2 cup medium white wine

- 1.5 cup water

- 16 each mussels

- 8 ounces shrimp (large)

- 8 ounces scallops (large)

- 1/4 cup garlic (fresh) chopped

- 1/2 cup shallots sliced

- 1 tablespoon thyme (fresh) piced & chopped

- 1/2 each fennel

- 4 each red peppers diced

- 4 cup peas

- 4 ounces tomato sauce, Pritikin

- 4 each cherry tomatoes

- 1/4 cup parley (fresh) chopped

- 1/4 cup tarragon-fresh

Instructions

- Saute shallot & garlic in a stockpot.

- Add rice when garlic is light brown.

- Cook for 30 seconds then add wine, fish stock & water.

- Bring to a boil and boil for 5 minutes.

- Lower heat and cover.

- Place in 350-degree oven for 40 minutes.

- When rice is cooked, in a large skillet saute remaining ingredients, except parsley & tarragon.

- When scallops & shrimp are cooked add rice & herbs.

- Mix well & serve.

Pritikin Brownie

Course: Dessert, Entertaining, Vegetarian

Cuisine: American, International, Vegetarian

Materials

- 1/4 cup canola oil (or apple sauce)

- 1/4 cup water warm

- 1/2 cup cocoa powder (unsweeted)

- 1/2 cup Splenda

- 2 teaspoons vanilla extract

- 1/4 cup egg whites

- 1/2 cup flour (whole wheat)

- 1/4 cup nuts chopped, or raisons

Instructions

• Pre-heat oven at 350 F

• Lightly grease an 8 inch square pan or line with greased paper

• In a medium bowl combine oil, water and cocoa powder and stir until cocoa powder is dissolved

• Add Splenda and mix well

• Add egg whites and stir until well combined

• Stir in vanilla. Add flour. Mix until all the flour is mixed in (do not over mix)

• Fold in nuts

• Spread in pan and bake for 25 minutes

• Cool completely before cutting into squares

Jambalaya

Course: Dinner, Lunch, Main Course, Main Dish, Soup/Stew, Vegetarian

Cuisine: Asian, Continental, Vegan, Vegetarian

Yield: 12 people

Materials

• 1 cup vegetable stock

• 1.5 green bell peppers chopped

• 1 large onion chopped

• 1 large tomato chopped

• 1 cup mixed fresh seasonal vegetables cut in chunks (I use frozen and it worked just fine)

• 2 pounds tofu

• 1 teaspoon salt

• 1/4 to 1/2 teaspoon cayenne pepper

• 8 cups brown rice cooked

• 1 cup tomato puree (low sodium)

• 1/2 cup carrot shredded

• 1/2 cup scallions chopped

• 1/2 cup broccoli

• 1/4 cup cauliflower

• 1/2 cup red pepper diced

• 3 tablespoons thyme (fresh)

• 1 teaspoon paprika

• 1 teaspoon chili powder

Instructions

• In medium pot over medium heat add stock, peppers, onion, tomato and cauliflower & broccoli.

• Simmer, stirring occasionally, until vegetables are tender, about 10 minutes.

• Add tofu and seasonings; cook 5 more minutes.

• Stir in rice and tomato puree; continue stirring until mixture is thoroughly blended.

• Serve hot garnished with carrot and scallions.

The Complete Pritikin Smoothie Recipes

Green Power Smoothie

Ingredients:

1. 1 cup spinach

2. 1/2 cucumber

3. 1 green apple

4. 1/2 avocado

5. 1 cup unsweetened almond milk

6. Juice of 1/2 lemon

Instructions:

1. Add the spinach, cucumber, green apple, and avocado to a blender.

2. Pour in the almond milk and lemon juice.

3. Blend until smooth. Serve immediately.

Berry Bliss Smoothie

Ingredients:

1. 1 cup mixed berries (strawberries, blueberries, raspberries)

2. 1/2 banana

3. 1 cup unsweetened almond milk

4. 1 tablespoon chia seeds

Instructions:

1. Combine the berries, banana, almond milk, and chia seeds in a blender.

2. Blend until smooth. Enjoy chilled.

Tropical Detox Smoothie

Ingredients:

1. 1 cup pineapple chunks

2. 1/2 banana

3. 1/2 cup coconut water

4. 1/2 cup spinach

5. 1/2 tablespoon flaxseeds

Instructions:

1. Place the pineapple, banana, coconut water, spinach, and flaxseeds in a blender.

2. Blend until smooth. Serve over ice.

Citrus Green Smoothie

Ingredients:

1. 1 orange, peeled

2. 1/2 grapefruit, peeled

3. 1 cup kale

4. 1/2 banana

5. 1 cup water

Instructions:

1. Add the orange, grapefruit, kale, banana, and water to a blender.

2. Blend until smooth. Drink fresh.

Avocado Berry Smoothie

Ingredients:

1. 1/2 avocado

2. 1/2 cup blueberries

3. 1/2 cup strawberries

4. 1 cup unsweetened almond milk

5. 1 tablespoon hemp seeds

Instructions:

1. Combine the avocado, blueberries, strawberries, almond milk, and hemp seeds in a blender.
2. Blend until creamy. Serve immediately.

Apple Cinnamon Smoothie

Ingredients:

1. 1 apple, cored and sliced

2. 1/2 banana

3. 1 cup unsweetened almond milk

4. 1 teaspoon cinnamon

5. 1 tablespoon chia seeds

Instructions:

1. Place the apple, banana, almond milk, cinnamon, and chia seeds in a blender.

2. Blend until smooth. Enjoy right away.

Peachy Green Smoothie

Ingredients:

1. 1 peach, pitted and sliced

2. 1/2 banana

3. 1 cup spinach

4. 1 cup water

5. 1 tablespoon flaxseeds

Instructions:

1. Add the peach, banana, spinach, water, and flaxseeds to a blender.

2. Blend until smooth. Drink fresh.

Mango Turmeric Smoothie

Ingredients:

1. 1 cup mango chunks

2. 1/2 banana

3. 1 cup unsweetened almond milk

4. 1/2 teaspoon turmeric

5. 1/2 teaspoon ginger

Instructions:

1. Combine the mango, banana, almond milk, turmeric, and ginger in a blender.
2. Blend until smooth. Serve immediately.

Blueberry Oat Smoothie

Ingredients:

1. 1/2 cup blueberries

2. 1/2 banana

3. 1/4 cup oats

4. 1 cup unsweetened almond milk

5. 1 tablespoon chia seeds

Instructions:

1. Place the blueberries, banana, oats, almond milk, and chia seeds in a blender.

2. Blend until smooth. Enjoy chilled.

Strawberry Kiwi Smoothie

Ingredients:

1. 1 cup strawberries

2. 1 kiwi, peeled

3. 1/2 banana

4. 1 cup unsweetened almond milk

5. 1 tablespoon flaxseeds

Instructions:

1. Add the strawberries, kiwi, banana, almond milk, and flaxseeds to a blender.

2. Blend until smooth. Drink fresh.

Carrot Ginger Smoothie

Ingredients:

1. 1 cup carrots, chopped

2. 1/2 banana1/2 inch piece of ginger

3. 1 cup unsweetened almond milk

4. 1 tablespoon chia seeds

Instructions:

1. Combine the carrots, banana, ginger, almond milk, and chia seeds in a blender.

2. Blend until smooth. Serve immediately.

Pineapple Spinach Smoothie

Ingredients:

1. 1 cup pineapple chunks

2. 1 cup spinach

3. 1/2 banana

4. 1 cup coconut water

Instructions:

1. Place the pineapple, spinach, banana, and coconut water in a blender.

2. Blend until smooth. Enjoy chilled.

Raspberry Almond Smoothie

Ingredients:

1. 1 cup raspberries

2. 1/2 banana

3. 1 cup unsweetened almond milk

4. 1 tablespoon almond butter

Instructions:

1. Add the raspberries, banana, almond milk, and almond butter to a blender.
2. Blend until smooth. Drink fresh.

Citrus Berry Smoothie

Ingredients:

1. 1 orange, peeled

2. 1/2 cup blueberries

3. 1/2 banana

4. 1 cup water

5. 1 tablespoon flaxseeds

Instructions:

1. Combine the orange, blueberries, banana, water, and flaxseeds in a blender.

2. Blend until smooth. Serve immediately.

Chocolate Banana Smoothie

Ingredients:

1. 1 banana

2. 1 tablespoon unsweetened cocoa powder

3. 1 cup unsweetened almond milk

4. 1 tablespoon chia seeds

Instructions:

1. Place the banana, cocoa powder, almond milk, and chia seeds in a blender.

2. Blend until smooth. Enjoy right away.

Green Detox Smoothie

Ingredients:

1. 1 cup kale

2. 1/2 cucumber

3. 1 green apple

4. 1/2 avocado

5. 1 cup water

6. Juice of 1/2 lemon

Instructions:

1. Add the kale, cucumber, apple, avocado, water, and lemon juice to a blender.

2. Blend until smooth. Drink fresh.

Strawberry Banana Smoothie

Ingredients:

1. 1 cup strawberries

2. 1 banana

3. 1 cup unsweetened almond milk

4. 1 tablespoon chia seeds

Instructions:

1. Combine the strawberries, banana, almond milk, and chia seeds in a blender.

2. Blend until smooth. Serve immediately.

Mango Spinach Smoothie

Ingredients:

1. 1 cup mango chunks

2. 1 cup spinach

3. 1/2 banana

4. 1 cup water

Instructions:

1. Place the mango, spinach, banana, and water in a blender.

2. Blend until smooth. Enjoy chilled.

Blueberry Kale Smoothie

Ingredients:

1. 1/2 cup blueberries

2. 1 cup kale

3. 1/2 banana

4. 1 cup unsweetened almond milk

5. 1 tablespoon flaxseeds

Instructions:

1. Add the blueberries, kale, banana, almond milk, and flaxseeds to a blender.

2. Blend until smooth. Drink fresh.

Pineapple Coconut Smoothie

Ingredients:

1. 1 cup pineapple chunks

2. 1/2 banana

3. 1/2 cup unsweetened coconut milk

4. 1/2 cup water

Instructions:

1. Combine the pineapple, banana, coconut milk, and water in a blender.

2. Blend until smooth. Serve immediately.

Apple Spinach Smoothie

Ingredients:

1. 1 apple, cored and sliced

2. 1 cup spinach

3. 1/2 banana

4. 1 cup unsweetened almond milk

5. 1 tablespoon chia seeds

Instructions:

1. Place the apple, spinach, banana, almond milk, and chia seeds in a blender.

2. Blend until smooth. Enjoy right away.

Peach Berry Smoothie

Ingredients:

1. 1 peach, pitted and sliced

2. 1/2 cup mixed berries

3. 1/2 banana

4. 1 cup unsweetened almond milk

Instructions:

1. Add the peach, berries, banana, and almond milk to a blender.

2. Blend until smooth. Serve immediately.

Carrot Mango Smoothie

Ingredients:

1. 1 cup carrots, chopped

2. 1 cup mango chunks

3. 1/2 banana

4. 1 cup water

Instructions:

1. Combine the carrots, mango, banana, and water in a blender.

2. Blend until smooth. Drink fresh.

Avocado Mint Smoothie

Ingredients:

1. 1/2 avocado

2. 1/2 cup spinach

3. 1/2 banana

4. 1 cup unsweetened almond milk

5. A few fresh mint leaves

Instructions:

1. Place the avocado, spinach, banana, almond milk, and mint leaves in a blender.

2. Blend until smooth. Enjoy chilled.

Snacks and Appetizers for Pritikin Diet

Hummus and Veggie Sticks

Ingredients:

1. Carrot sticks, cucumber slices, bell pepper strips

2. Homemade hummus (made with chickpeas, lemon juice, garlic, and tahini)

Instructions:

1. Wash and cut vegetables into sticks or slices.

2. Serve with a side of homemade hummus for dipping.

Greek Yogurt with Berries

Ingredients:

1. Plain Greek yogurt (low-fat or non-fat)

2. Mixed berries (strawberries, blueberries, raspberries)

Instructions:

1. Spoon Greek yogurt into a bowl.

2. Top with fresh berries for added fiber and antioxidants.

Avocado Toast on Whole Grain Bread

Ingredients:

1. Whole grain bread, toasted

2. Ripe avocado, mashed

3. Sliced tomatoes

4. Sprinkle of black pepper and sea salt

Instructions:

1. Spread mashed avocado evenly on toasted bread slices.

2. Top with sliced tomatoes, black pepper, and a pinch of sea salt.

Mixed Nuts and Seeds

Ingredients:

1. Almonds, walnuts, pistachios, pumpkin seeds, sunflower seeds

Instructions:

1. Mix nuts and seeds together in a bowl.

2. Portion into small servings for a quick, nutrient-dense snack.

Edamame Salad

Ingredients:

1. Steamed edamame beans

2. Diced cucumber

3. Cherry tomatoes, halved

4. Fresh parsley, chopped

5. Lemon juice and a drizzle of olive oil

Instructions:

1. Combine edamame, cucumber, tomatoes, and parsley in a bowl.

2. Dress with lemon juice and olive oil. Mix well before serving.

Baked Sweet Potato Fries

Ingredients:

1. Sweet potatoes, cut into fries

2. Olive oil spray

3. Paprika, garlic powder, sea salt

Instructions:

1. Preheat oven to 400°F (200°C).

2. Toss sweet potato fries with olive oil spray and seasonings.

3. Bake for 20-25 minutes until crispy. Serve hot.

Caprese Skewers

Ingredients:

1. Cherry tomatoes

2. Fresh basil leaves

3. Mozzarella cheese balls (part-skim)

4. Balsamic glaze (optional)

Instructions:

1. Thread cherry tomatoes, basil leaves, and mozzarella balls onto skewers.

2. Drizzle with balsamic glaze if desired. Serve chilled.

Chia Seed Pudding

Ingredients:

1. Chia seeds

2. Unsweetened almond milk

3. Vanilla extract

4. Fresh berries for topping

Instructions:

1. Mix chia seeds, almond milk, and vanilla extract in a bowl.

2. Refrigerate overnight until thickened.

3. Top with fresh berries before serving.

Quinoa Salad Cups

Ingredients:

1. Cooked quinoa

2. Diced cucumbers, bell peppers, cherry tomatoes

3. Lemon juice, olive oil, fresh herbs (like parsley or cilantro)

Instructions:

1. Combine quinoa and chopped vegetables in a bowl.

2. Dress with lemon juice, olive oil, and herbs.

3. Serve in small cups for easy portion control.

Stuffed Bell Peppers

Ingredients:

1. Bell peppers, halved and seeded

2. Quinoa and vegetable stuffing (sauteed onions, spinach, mushrooms)

3. Low-fat shredded cheese (optional)

Instructions:

1. Preheat oven to 375°F (190°C).

2. Stuff bell pepper halves with quinoa and vegetable mixture.

3. Top with a sprinkle of low-fat cheese and bake for 20-25 minutes.

7 Days Meal plan for Weight Loss

Week 1

Day 1:

1. Breakfast: Oatmeal with fresh berries and a sprinkle of chia seeds.

2. Lunch: Mixed green salad with grilled chicken breast and a side of quinoa.

3. Dinner: Baked salmon with steamed broccoli and brown rice.

4. Snack: Carrot sticks with hummus.

Day 2:

1. Breakfast: Greek yogurt topped with sliced banana and a drizzle of honey.

2. Lunch: Whole grain wrap with turkey, avocado, spinach, and tomato.

3. Dinner: Stir-fried tofu with mixed vegetables and brown rice.

4. Snack: Handful of mixed nuts.

Day 3:

1. Breakfast: Smoothie with spinach, berries, banana, and almond milk.

2. Lunch: Lentil soup with a side of mixed green salad.

3. Dinner: Grilled shrimp skewers with quinoa and steamed asparagus.

4. Snack: Apple slices with almond butter.

Day 4:

1. Breakfast: Whole grain toast topped with mashed avocado and poached eggs.

2. Lunch: Chickpea salad with cucumber, cherry tomatoes, and lemon vinaigrette.

3. Dinner: Grilled chicken breast with roasted sweet potatoes and green beans.

4. Snack: Edamame beans.

Day 5:

1. Breakfast: Chia seed pudding with fresh berries.

2. Lunch: Whole wheat pasta primavera with marinara sauce and side salad.

3. Dinner: Baked cod with quinoa pilaf and steamed broccoli.

4. Snack: Greek yogurt with sliced almonds.

Day 6:

1. Breakfast: Smoothie with mango, spinach, banana, and coconut water.

2. Lunch: Black bean and corn salad with avocado and lime dressing.

3. Dinner: Turkey meatballs in marinara sauce with zucchini noodles.

4. Snack: Cottage cheese with pineapple chunks.

Day 7:

1. Breakfast: Whole grain pancakes topped with fresh berries and a dollop of Greek yogurt.

2. Lunch: Grilled vegetable wrap with hummus on whole wheat tortilla.

3. Dinner: Quinoa-stuffed bell peppers with side salad.

4. Snack: Mixed berries with a sprinkle of granola.

CONCLUSION

The Pritikin Diet is a great option for those who want to lose weight and improve their health. It is a low-fat, high-fiber diet that promotes the consumption of whole, natural foods. By following the Pritikin Diet, you can improve your heart health, control diabetes, lower blood pressure, reduce the risk of cancer, and promote weight loss. Additionally, since the Pritikin Diet is based on healthy eating principles, it is a sustainable and effective option for long-term weight loss and health improvement.